Fermented Drinks and Condiments

Why You Should Consume Fermented Foods

Table of Contents

Introduction

I want to thank you and congratulate you for downloading the book on Fermented Drinks and Condiments.

This book contains proven steps on how fermented drinks and condiments are good for your health as well as different recipes for different fermented drinks and condiments. You will also learn about different resources that you can use to further your education on fermentation and the process.

Here's an inescapable fact: you will learn about the fermentation process that has proven to help improve your health! Not only that, but you will gain a new knowledge of some recipes on how you can make your own fermented food or drinks.

If you do not develop your knowledge on the different ways that fermentation is actually good for you, then this book has not done its job. Hopefully the resources used in this book will help to engage you into a new world of fermentation and possibly get you to change your diet to include some of these awesome recipes that you can introduce not only to your family, but your friends as well.

It's time for you to learn and become an amazing expert on fermentation and the benefits that it has. You may be surprised about the information that this book contains. You will be able to find additional resources that will help you learn additional information that you may need in order to begin your journey with fermentation.

Note: If you are allergic to anything listed in any of the recipes that is used for the fermentation, please do not consume it. If you have any health issues that concern you as to if you should consume anything that has been fermented (outside of alcohol) please consult your doctor before consumption.

Chapter One: What is Fermentation?

Fermentation is a process in which the metabolic system converts any sugars into acids, alcohol, or gases. This mostly occurs in things such as yeast, bacteria, and any oxygen-starved muscle cells.

This can also be a broader explanation as to the bulk growth of microorganisms based on their growth medium while producing specific chemical products. The French microbiologist Louis Pasteur is actually the one who is most often credited for the insights that helped with our knowledge on fermentation and its microbial causes.

Since the Neolithic times, fermentation has been used, especially in beverages. Documents with fermentation have been dated back to 7000-6600 BCE in Jiahu, China. In India, medicated wines have been documented as using the fermentation process as well as foods being fermented during the Ancient Egyptian, Babylonian, Sudan, and even pre-Hispanic Mexico.

These fermented foods have been used in Judaism and Christianity. The god of fermentation is actually known as the Baltic god Rugutis.

Three publications appeared by C. Cagniard de la Tour, T. Swann, and F. Kuetzing during the years 1837-1838 on yeast and how it is a living organism that reproduces by budding. Foods such as beer, wine, and bread were basic foods in Europe and any early investigations on fermentation were done with yeast as they were made.

Once bacteria was discovered, it was first coined in English during the 1840s however did not become used until the 1870s which then was connected with the new germ theory of disease.

During the 1850s and 60s Louis Pasteur proved that fermentation was first initiated by living organisms. It wasn't until 1857 that Pasteur was able to prove that lactic acid fermentation was also caused by living organisms. However, he was able to demonstrate that bacteria is what caused milk to sour which was formerly thought to only be a chemical change. His work on identifying the role of the microorganisms in food spoilage helped to lead to the process of pasteurization.

Some traditional uses for fermentation were to be able to enrich the diet of a person through the development of the diversity of flavors, aromas, and textures of food. It also helped to eliminate any antinutrients along with decreasing the cooking time therefore decreasing the fuel required to cook the food. Fermentation also helped to preserve substantial amounts of food by using lactic acid, acetic acid, alcohol, as well as alkaline fermentation. In addition to that, foods were enriched with proteins, vitamins, and essential amino acids.

Foods were and are also fermented by the region in which they come from. Some of the world wide foods that are fermented are things we know as cheese, bread, yogurt, olives, vinegar, wine, and alcohol.

Such as with anything, there are some risks when it comes to consuming fermented foods and drinks. Since 1985, the state of Alaska has been witness to an increase of botulism cases. Along with Alaska, there are other states that see this, but this is the state that has seen the most cases.

It is believed that this is caused because of the traditional practice of allowing animal products to ferment for extended periods of time before they are consumed. This practice was and is practiced by the Eskimo's with foods such as birds, seal oil, beaver tails, whale flippers, sea lions, walrus, fish heads as well as whole fish.

The risk of botulism is also present when placing food into a plastic container for storage. The botulinum bacteria tends to thrive when the anaerobic conditions are created by any air tight environment that can be achieved by plastic.

The World Health Organization has since classified any pickled foods possibly containing carcinogenic by product called ethyl carbamate (urethane). Back in 2009, there was a review that has shown regularly consuming pickled vegetables can roughly double a person's risk for esophageal squamous cell carcinoma.

Chapter Two: The Health Benefits of Fermentation

There are several great health benefits when it comes to both fermented drinks and fermented foods. While each drink and food has its own health benefits, there are some benefits that all foods and drinks will have that have been fermented.

Fermented foods will help with probiotics as they introduce beneficial bacteria into your digestive system therefore helping to balance the bacteria in your digestive system. Probiotics have also been proven to help with bowel health, improve your immunity, slow or even reverse some diseases.

You will also be able to absorb food better. Once your body has the proper balance of bacteria you will have enough digestive enzymes that will help your body to absorb the nutrients in foods that your body needs. Because of this, your body will no longer need as many supplements and vitamins that you may have been taking in order to replace anything that your body has been missing.

As you will begin to see a common thread appears when it comes to the actual benefits of fermented foods and drinks and that is that there is an added benefit when it comes to helping your abdominal health along with an increased vitamin content.

Many of the fermented foods and drinks have shown that they have helped to benefit diseases such as cancer and arthritis. Do not replace any medications that your doctor has given you to help combat any illness with fermented foods because you believe that they will cure you. There is no proven studies that show that they will actually cure anything.

So, now that we know about some of the basic health benefits, let's look more closely at some of the health benefits of specific fermented drinks and foods.

Fermented Coconut Water: Coconut kefir comes with every benefit that raw coconut water has but there are the extra benefits that come from the fermentation process. Being that it is sugar-free, it is a great drink for anyone who has diabetes or several other advanced illnesses.

During the fermentation process, the coconut water may become slightly sour but then eventually sweet and fizzy much like a champagne beverage.

Additional health benefits are that it is a good source of probiotics. Probiotics as we've mentioned help with the bacteria in your gut and improve your immune system. Two ounces of fermented coconut water can actually contain up to 200 trillion cells of healthy bacteria.

It can also help with any bloating that you may be experiencing therefore flattening your stomach. At the time boating occurs, it means that your intestines are inflamed therefore meaning that food is not being fully digested causing the stomach to appear larger than it truly is. The coconut water can actually help to sooth the intestines and improve your digestion.

Along with these, you will also discover that you will experience blemishes, scaring, pigmentation, and acne fading should you digest it regularly. Along with this, you will discover your hair appears to be healthier, your moods being more balanced as well as having more energy.

Fermented coconut water is just regular coconut water that has been through the fermentation process obviously, but with the fermentation process you will discover that you gain some health benefits that you did not previously have when it came to drinking regular coconut water.

Beet Kvass: Fermented beet kvass can actually help to lower your blood pressure. There is a "secret" ingredient called nitrate that helps to lower blood pressure. At the point of conversion from nitrates to nitric oxide, it can be absorbed into the blood stream.

Nitric oxide helps to save people who use nitro-glycerine when they begin to feel the symptoms of heart attacks.

The additional resources of fermented beet kvass are that you will get antioxidents as well as fiber, iron, folate (B-vitamin), vitamin C, manganese, copper, and potassium.

Kefir: this is much like coconut water but made with grains, you are able to make it with fruit as well or milk.

The health benefits of kefir include: a probiotic rich substance that can help you with your digestive health (just like every other drink that we have discussed). Probiotics will help to eliminate the harmful bacteria that makes its home inside your digestive tract.

Kefir has also been proven to help those that are suffering from diabetes as well as those that are lactose intolerant. The grains that are used to make kefir are actually made of bacteria that eats at sugar as well as lactose which will remove the sugar from the body before it can flood your bloodstream and cause the all too harmful spikes/plunges in blood sugar that diabetics need to avoid in order to remain healthy.

The lactose eating bacteria can also help to keep your stomach from getting violently upset like it will when you digest anything that has lactose. So, without having to deal with the sickness, you are still able to get the nutrients that your body needs from milk.

Kefiran that we find present in the kefir has actually been shown to help suppress a person's blood pressure as well as to reduce the serum cholesterol. With reduced cholesterol and a lowered blood pressure you will find that your heart will be healthier than it has been and therefore you will be less prone to such conditions as heart attacks, strokes, and atherosclerosis.

Please note that just because you are drinking kefir does not mean that you are not going to possibly have a heart attack, stroke, or other heart conditions. It is important that you talk with your doctor to make sure that you are not harming yourself by drinking this fermented drink.

So, along with the very rich source of protein you will find in kefir, you will also see your organ functions increase as well as a boost in your metabolism. An added bonus is that you will see your wounds healing better as well as the time it takes for you to recover decreasing so that it does not take as long for you to recover. Let's not forget that it helps to promote cellular growth!

Remember that no natural dangers have been shown to occur while drinking kefir, you may notice that you have an increased number of trips to the bathroom because it is helping to clean the toxins out of your system.

Kombucha: Kombucha is known in ancient China as the "immortal health elixir," that has proven benefits of helping to prevent and fight arthritis, cancer, as well as several other degenerative diseases.

This tea is actually fermented by using bacteria and yeast.

One of the health benefits of drinking fermented kombucha is that it can help to detox your body. The process of detoxification can actually help to produce healthy livers as well as aid in cancer prevention. While drinking kombucha, your body will ease the load that is placed on your liver.

Because of how high the kombucha is in glucaric acide, it has been shown to help prevent cancer based on recent studies.

Along with helping to prevent cancer, the glucosamines have been proven to help prevent as well as treat all the different forms of arthritis. Therefore, the pain in your joints will lessen and give you the relief that NSAIDs may have been giving you before. Without joint pain, you will realize more flexibility and even reduce wrinkles.

Additionally, you will notice a difference in your digestion and gut health. Due to the colony of bacteria and yeast that helps to ferment kombucha it is an excellent source of probiotics.

Thus, you may notice a reduced or even completely vanished symptoms that you see from anxiety, depression and fibromyalgia.

Health benefits don't just come from fermented drinks though. There are also added health benefits that you can receive when it comes to fermented foods.

Sauerkraut: As you may know, sauerkraut usually comes in a can or jar and is something that you use as a hot dog topping. There aren't many people who enjoy it because of the smell or even the taste.

However, those of us that actually enjoy sauerkraut will be interested in finding out that there are health benefits that come with adding this delicious topping

Just like we've discovered with most fermented foods and drinks, there are probiotics that help to assist in abdominal health. But, along with that, you will discover that sauerkraut is a good source of vitamin C. Back when people would travel across the ocean on long voyages, sauerkraut was taken so that they could combat vitamin C deficiency.

Like many things we've already talked about, sauerkraut also has some properties that help to fight cancer. It is found that through the fermentation process isothiocyanates help to prohibit the growth of cancer. It has also been found that the glucosinolates help to activate what the body naturally produces such as antioxidant enzymes.

Ulcers have also been treated with sauerkraut. This is traditionally a practice that is found in European countries. Because the cabbage is a source of vitamin U, it is used to help treat the peptic ulcers some people suffer from.

So perhaps much like an apple a day keeps the doctor away, perhaps a serving of sauerkraut a day will keep the ulcers away!

Pickles: Pickles, who doesn't love them? We eat them plan, on our hamburgers, in our food, they are or can be put in almost everything. But again, what are the health benefits of fermented pickles?

Just like it seems everything that is fermented, it is an excellent source of probiotics in which will help to improve the immune system functions as well as intestinal tract health. Add in that it can decrease allergies and protect against microbial infections.

You will also see reduced flu and cold symptoms that you would normally go get antibiotics for. They may even help to reduce a person's risk of colon cancer.

When looking at recent studies, it has been found that gut microbiota will communicate with the central nervous system to help improve brain functions and behaviors such as pain, cognition, mood, and anxiety.

So, just looking at a few of the health benefits of fermented drinks and food, it seems to be proven that fermented foods and drinks are just better for our health than we thought it was. Maybe it is more efficient that we switch our diets and include more fermentation to help us improve the functions of our body as well as help to prevent certain diseases.

Chapter Three: Fermented Condiments

Condiments, we love them and we hate them. Things like sauerkraut, pickles, kimchi, and other condiments can be an acquired taste or something that we grow up loving. It all depends on what we like and how we were raised that depends on if we prefer condiments.

But, some condiments can be fermented to not only give us added health benefits, but can also enhance the taste of the food. Once again, this is a preference that is based on the person who is eating the condiment.

In this chapter, we will explore how certain fermented foods are made as well as a recipe to help you discover if you like this food or not. Do not be discouraged if you find that you do not like a certain food fermented. The fermentation process can actually end up changing how a food tastes due to the vinegar in which most foods are fermented in.

Sauerkraut:

Like we've mentioned before, sauerkraut is a food that is very high in vitamin C. It is something that not everyone will like obviously, but what isn't that way?

A process called lactic acid fermentation is what is normally used to ferment sauerkraut as well as several other foods that are fermented. The cabbage (whether red or white) is finely shredded then a layer of salt is added to it before being left alone.

Normally the fermentation process takes several months as the sauerkraut is left in an airtight container. Pasteurization or refrigeration is not a required step in this process however, adding them to the process can help to prolong the storage life of the sauerkraut.

Lactobacilli is introduced into the air born bacteria on the raw cabbage where when left will grow. The yeast that is present could be the reason that some of the sauerkraut ends up yielding poor flavored sauerkraut because the temperature of where the cabbage is stored is too high.

Ultimately, there are three phases to the fermentation process. The first phase is when the anaerobic bacteria leads to the fermentation and begins to provide the proper environment that the bacteria will later prefer. The second phase happens as the acid levels grow and certain types of bacteria begin to take dominance over the environment around them. Lastly, the remaining sugars begin to ferment and the pH levels are lowered.

If the sauerkraut has been cured properly, then it is acidic enough to prevent an environment that is favorable for the growth of the toxins that can cause botulism.

Recipe for Sauerkraut:

- 1 apple, peeled and diced (optional)
- 1 28 oz can sauerkraut
- 3 juniper berries or 1 tsp caraway seeds (optional)
- 1 onion chopped

- 1-2 tbsp cornstarch
- 1-2 tbsp oil, butter, or bacon drippings
- 2/3 cup liquid (broth, apple juice, water, white wine)
- Salt, pepper, sugar

Drain sauerkraut getting as much liquid out as possible.

Heat the oil in the frying pan

Add in the onions and sauté them until golden

Once golden, add sauerkraut and continue to brown. If necessary, add extra oil

If you are using juniper berries, caraway seeds, or even apple, add it in here.

Add some additional liquid and bring to a simmer

Cover the pan and cook for about fifteen minutes but no longer than an hour. Stir occasionally adding additional liquid if necessary.

With cold water, mix in cornstarch and add to the sauerkraut but only add enough to thicken the sauce

Season with your salt, pepper, and sugar

Cucumber Pickles

Making cucumber pickles is actually fairly easy. You take a cucumber and ferment it much like you did with the sauerkraut but in something such as vinegar or another solution that will help to aid in the fermentation process. Just like with the sauerkraut, you're going to leave the jar alone for an extended period of time to allow the bacteria time to do its job.

- 4 garlic cloves, thinly sliced
- 6 cups thinly sliced pickling cucumbers
- ¼ tsp freshly ground black pepper
- 2 cups thinly sliced onion
- ½ tsp crushed red pepper
- ¾ cup of sugar
- ½ tsp ground turmeric
- ¾ tsp salt
- ½ tsp celery seeds
- ½ tsp mustard seeds
- 1 ½ cup white vinegar

You're going to place about three cups of cucumbers into a glass bowl

Top with the onion

Repeat process until all is in the bowl

Combine vinegar and all other ingredients into saucepan

Bring to a boil and stir well.

Cook for an additional minute

Pour over cucumber mix

Let cool

Chill and cover for about four days.

Note: the pickles may be stored in the fridge for up to a month

Kimchi

It should come as no big surprise when I tell you that kimchi is made much like the sauerkraut and cucumber pickles are.

For traditional preparations, the kimichi should be stored underground so that they can be kept cool in the summer as well as warm in the winter.

Kimchi can be made from things such as cabbage, scallions, cucumbers, and even radishes.

Much like sauerkraut you're going to place the ingredients in the salt water for about eight hours. Once the time is up, you're going to rinse them off and place them in a bowl to add any spices that you wish to have in it. Spices can be things like ginger, garlic and even red pepper flakes. If you're wanting something a little sweeter, add in some soy sauce or sugar.

After you've done this, place into a food safe container making sure you place enough brine in the container to ensure that the vegetables are covered. It is important that you try and keep the vegetables from floating to the surface.

Check to ensure that the vegetables are still covered in brine as well as removing any white film that could grow on top of it. Once two weeks have passed, your kimchi will be done.

Kimchi Pancakes

- Oil
- 1 cup chopped kimchi

- ½ cup of all-purpose flour
- 3 tbsp kimchi juice
- ½ tsp sugar
- ¼ cup water
- ½ tsp salt
- 2 tbsp chopped onion

Mix all ingredients together except for the oil

Heat in a flat bottom, non-stick skillet a generous amount of oil

Place batter in the pan (it will make a sizzle sound)

Spread over the pan and cook until the bottom is brown and crispy

Flip and repeat.

Turn down the heat and flip once more to ensure it is cooked thoroughly

Allow to cool before cutting into bite sized pieces and serving

Fermented Salsa

Since salsa includes many different ingredients you won't find a "traditional" fermentation process. Each of the ingredients will be added into the salsa and the salsa as a whole will be fermented thus causing all the ingredients to ferment at once.

Salsa as everyone knows can be used for things such as burritos, tacos, and various other foods as well as making it as a dip. This salsa (from personal experience) will tend to be slightly runnier than the traditional salsas because of the fermentation process. This however does not detract from the actual taste of the salsa.

- 1 lrg onion or a bunch of green onions cut into large chunks
- ¼-1/2 cup water
- 3 small bell peppers cored and cut into lrg chunks
- ½ cup whey
- 6 large garlic cloves peeled
- ¼-1/2 tsp cayenne powder
- ½ cup packed cilantro leaves unchopped
- 3 tbsp coarse celtic sea salt
- 2.5 lbs roma tomatoes cut into quarters
- Juice from 1 lemon

Combine the peppers, garlic and cilantro in your food processor pulse three to five times until everything is coarsely chopped

Add 1/3 of the tomatoes and pulse two to three more times until you've made room for more tomatoes.

Repeat until all the tomatoes are in there

Pulse for an addition three to five times to make sure all is chopped.

Pour contents into a large bowl

Add lemon juice, sea salt, whey, cayenne powder and stir

Wash jars with soap and hot water

Ladle salsa into jar leaving two to three inches of head space

Add water to submerge salsa

Close lid tightly and leave alone for a few days until you see bubbles

Stir if vegetables have separated from liquid until redisbursed and submerged

Transfer to cold storage.

Fermented Fruit Chutney

Once again, you will find that this recipe does not call for you to ferment anything individually. The entire process will ferment the whole recipe leaving you with a delicious treat to share with your friends and family or even keep to yourself.

- ½ cup filtered water
- ½ tsp caraway seeds
- 2 tbsp whey
- ½ tsp dried thyme
- 2 tbsp honey
- ½ tsp ground spicebush berries or black pepper
- 1 tbsp vinegar
- ½ tsp red pepper flakes (or more should you like it spicy)
- 3 cups peeled cored and finely chopped apples or other fruit of your choice
- 1 tsp slightly crushed coriander seeds
- ½ cup raisins or small pieces of other dried fruit
- 1 tsp ground cumin
- 2 tsp sea salt

Combine the water, vinegar, honey and whey

Mix other ingredients and pack firmly into jar leaving at least an inch of head space.

Liquid needs to come to the top of the fruit, if it doesn't add a little less filtered water

Cover and leave at room temperature for at least two days

Refrigerate and leave for another week before opening

Will keep in the fridge for about two months.

Chapter Four: Fermented Drinks

We've talked about the health benefits of fermented drinks just like we had with the fermented condiments. But, once again that leaves us wondering how they are made and how we can make them ourselves.

In this chapter we will once again explore how some fermented drinks are made as well as a recipe for each of them.

Fermented Coconut Water

Making fermented coconut water is fairly simple. You're actually going to take your regular coconut water and warm it up to about 100 degrees. Once you've done this, you will then place it into your fermenting jar and add a probiotic (a small package you can buy) in for starter.

If you're doing twelve ounces of water, you will approximately use ¼ of a teaspoon of probiotic. Then you will mix with a spoon and place the lid on it. Place it in a warm location and wrap something around the jar in order to keep the light out.

On average you will have to wait three days for your coconut water to ferment. You will know if it is ready should you see that the water has started to bubble. There should also be a thin layer or white foam on the top and your water will have turned cloudy. Beware though because it will have a vinegar tang followed by that sweet coconut aftertaste.

Coconut water vinaigrette:

- ¼ cup coconut water
- ½ tsp black pepper
- 2 tbsp fresh lemon juice
- 1 tsp sea salt
- 2 tbsp olive oil

Add all ingredients together and let sit for a little while before adding to your favorite salad.

Kefir

There are different types of kefir that you can make. Kefir can be made from both milk and water. You can also make kefir with your own grains or using powder packets. It is truly up to you on how you want to make it.

What you're going to do you'll be placing your kefir grains and milk into your jar and covering it tightly before setting out in a room that is room temperature for up to twenty-four hours. Do not place in direct sunlight!

Make sure you shake the bottle a few times after fermentation to release any CO_2 gas that has built up.

You'll know when the fermentation progress is done when the grains have coagulated near the top of the jar.

Chipotle Avocado Kefir Sauce

- 2 very ripe large avocados
- 1/4-1/2 tsp ground chipotle powder
- ½-1 cup milk kefir (as needed to thin)
- 2 tsp apple cider vinegar
- 1/2-1tsp sea salt

Cut avocados in half and scoop out the soft flesh into a bowl

Mash with a fork

Add sea salt and vinegar before mixing well

Pour milk kefir in starting at ½ cup

Add until the mixture is thinned (even thinner if you're making salad dressing or thicker for dips)

Add chipotle powder until desired spiciness is reached

Kvass

Kvass is actually made from the fermentation of breads such as rye, wheat, or barley. It can be seasoned with fruit such as berries or raisins. Or, should you not want to do that, you can add in some birch sap.

Usually homemade kvass will be made using regular or black rye bread that has been dried and baked into croutons or fried with sugars or fruit. Yeast will be added in order to help with the fermentation process.

Kvass is normally served unfiltered and still has yeast in it.

Easy Bread Kvas

- 2.5 gallons of water
- 3 large plastic soda bottles
- 1lb of dark rye bread
- 5 tbsp dry yeast
- 1 handful raisins
- 4 cups sugar

Fill stock pot with water and bring to boil

Toast bread slices in toaster on the darkest setting

Once water is boiling, remove from heat

Add in raisins and bread

Cover and let sit overnight or at least for eight hours

Remove toast bread and discard

Mix sugar and yeast

Add into Kvass

Cover and leave for another six hours stirring occasionally

Discard raisins

Use cheese cloth to place Kvass into bottles

Close tightly and leave in fridge overnight.

Beet Kvass

Beet Kvass is the same as normal Kvass except it uses beets. It is made almost the same way, but there are a few differences that you will notice due to the fact you're using beets and not just normal kvass.

- 2-4 beets
- Half gallon glass jar
- ¼ cup whey or juice from sauerkraut
- Filtered water
- 1 tbsp sea salt or Himalayan salt

Wash beets and peel

Chop beets into small cubes (do not grate)

Place beets in bottom of jar

Add whey, juice, and salt

Fill jar with filtered water

Cover and leave for about two days

Transfer to the fridge after two days

Consume as desired

Kombucha

As mentioned earlier kombucha is a tea that most likely originated in ancient China, however that can*not be proved. It has the health benefits that we have talked about earlier and can also be consumed either every day or as you feel.

It is important to know that just like with anything, there are going to be dangers when it comes to consuming kombucha. Should you be concerned if you're supposed to be consuming it, please consult your doctor as well as do your research.

- Glass jar (quart or gallon)
- Rubber band
- Paper coffee filter
- Stirring utensil
- Unfluoridated and unchlorinated water
- Active kombucha scoby
- Distilled white vinegar
- Tea bags
- White sugar

Combine hot water and sugar in the jar make sure to stir until the sugar dissolves

Place your tea bags in the sugar water allowing them to steep

Cool your mixture down to about sixty-five degrees

Remove the tea bags

Add in your vinegar

Add in the active kombucha scoby

Cover and secure the filter with a rubber band

Allow to sit for about thirty days

Pour kombucha off the top of the jar and consume

Make sure to retain the scoby and enough liquid in the bottom of the jar so you can start a new batch

You can flavor your finished kombucha to taste

Chapter Five: Where to get them

If you're interested in more resources on how to go about fermenting different foods or drinks as well as how you can get these amazing recipes and many more both online and offline, there are some resources down below that can help you in your process.

Online

Weston A Price Foundation-information on Lacto-Fermentation

http://www.westonaprice.org/health-topics/lacto-fermentation/

National Center for Home Food Preservation-Safety tips on fermentation

www.nchpf.uga.edu/index.html

The FoxFire Book (ebook)

www.outpost-of-freedom.com/library/FoxfireVol1.pdf

Phickle- recipes with fermented drinks and foods as well as tips and experiences from those who consume or make fermented drinks and foods

www.phickle.com

Making Fermented Pickles and Sauerkraut- How to ferment pickles and sauerkraut

www.extension.umn.edu/food/food-safety/preserving/pickling/making-fermented-pickles-and-sauerkraut

Wild Fermentation- Workshops, recipes, articles and more on fermentation

www.wildfermentation.com

UGA Libraries-Books from the UGA Library that you can check out and read (additional books will be found below)

www.gil.find.uga.edu

Journals at UGA Libraries- journals you can read about fermentation (any non UGA journals can only be accessed on the UGA campus)

www.libs.uga.edu/ejournals

Books from Athens-Clarke Public- Additional books on Fermentation (books can be found below)

www.athenslibrary.org

CSU Frequently Asked Questions on fermentation

http://www.fshn.chhs.colostate.edu/students/undergraduate/fermentation-science/faqs.aspx

Important Facts as to why fermentation is good for us

http://www.treelight.com/health/nutrition/Fermentation.html

Yeast Strains

https://byo.com/resources/yeast

Cultured Food Classes-a website that will help you with cooking fermented foods as well as giving you additional resources via websites, books, and articles

http://cultured-foods.com/resources/

Offline

The Art of Fermentation: An In-Depth Exploration of Essential Concepts and Processes from Around the World by Sandor Ellix Katz

Wild Fermentation: The Flavor, Nutrition, and Craft of Live-Culture Foods by Sandor Ellix Katz

Wild Fermentation: A Do-It-Yourself Guide to Cultural Manipulation by Sandor Ellix Katz

Fermentation Workshop (DVD) by Sandor Katz

The Revolution Will Not Be Microwaved by Sandor Ellix Katz

The Enigma of Ferment: From the Philosopher's Stone to the First Biochemicle Nobel Price QR262.L22 2005 Science Library 4th Floor (on campus)

Fermented Fruits and Vegetables: A Global Perspective Folio QR115.B388 1998 Science Library 4th Floor (on campus)

The Oxford Handbook of Food Fermentations TP371.44.O94 2014 Science Library 4th Floor (on campus)

Cooked: A Natural History of Transformation Y10429 Main Library 1st Floor (on campus)

Pickled, Potted, and Canned: How the Art and Science of Food Preserving Changed the World

TX601.S47 2001 Science Library 3rd Floor (on campus)

Picked a Pickle: 50 Recipes for Pickles, Relishes, and Fermented Snacks NonFic 641.81 Acheson

Asian Pickles: Sweet, Sour, Salty, Cured, and Fermented Preserves from Korea, Japan, China, India, and Beyond NonFic 641.462 Solomon

Pickled, Potted, and Canned: How the Art and Science of Food Preserving Changed the World NonFic 641.4 Shepard

Nourishing Traditions: The Cookbook that Challenges Politically Correct Nutrition and the Diet Dictocrats by Sally Fallon and Mary Enig

The Essential Book of Fermentation: Great Taste and Good Health with Probiotic Foods by Jeff Cox

Conclusion

Thank you again for downloading this book! It is greatly appreciated!

I hope this book was able to help you to learn how the processes of fermentation not only is useful, but beneficial to your health.

The next step is to try and ferment your own food or drink of your choice. There are plenty of websites that offer recipes that you can use to try and ferment what you wish. As you may have realized, most of the fermentation process is the same for everything. Just add some vinegar and allow it to sit for several days or weeks. (Please remember that this process is not the absolute same for everything and that you need to find the proper process for fermentation based on what you're trying to ferment.)

Finally, if you enjoyed this book, take the time to share your thoughts and post a review on Amazon or the other major retailers website in which you purchased the book. It'd be much appreciated!

Thank you and good luck!